PROACTIVE APPROACHES ON ILEOSTOMY DIETING

Complete Low Residue, Low Fiber Ileostomy Diet Cookbook, Food & Recipes To Prevent Stoma Blockage, Decrease Swelling, Promote Digestion And Nourishment

DR. CHARLSE BLESSING

DISCLAIMER

The information in this book is meant solely for educational reasons. This book's contents are not meant to be used in place of expert medical advice, diagnosis, or treatment. Any decisions you make about your health must be discussed with a licensed healthcare provider.

Every effort has been made by the author to guarantee that the material in this book is correct and current as of the date of publication. Still, since medical knowledge advances rapidly, new studies might be conducted that change our understanding this illness and how best to manage it with food.

This book may contains references to and mentions of various people, things, websites, organizations, and other entities that the author does not support, advocate, or have any association with. There is no implied sponsorship or collaboration; all references and remarks are made only for informational purposes.

In order to address their individual health concerns, readers are advised to independently verify any information contained in this book and to consult with healthcare specialists. Any negative effects arising from the use or implementation of the material in this book, whether direct or indirect, are not the responsibility of the author or the publisher.

The dietary suggestions and counsel provided in this book are broad in scope and might not be appropriate for every individual. Readers are recommended to seek tailored counsel from trained healthcare specialists as individual health problems and demands differ.

The reader accepts the conditions of this disclaimer by reading this book.

FACTS ABOUT THIS BOOK

"Proactive Approaches on Ileostomy Dieting" is a vital resource for anyone navigating life after ileostomy surgery. This book starts with a thorough introduction to ileostomy, explaining the nuances of the surgical technique and stressing how important food is to the healing process. The foundation of this book is an understanding of the fundamentals of nutrition and digestion, as it explores the complexities of the digestive system and describes the dietary requirements unique to ileostomy patients.

The author carefully dissects the vital nutrients needed for the best possible health following an ileostomy, covering everything from proteins, carbs, and fats to a thorough examination of the vitamins and minerals that are vital for healing. Beyond generalizations, this book provides helpful guidance on customizing diet regimens to meet specific needs, along with a contemplative analysis of foods to include and exclude. The topic of hydration—which is sometimes disregarded—is discussed in detail, along with methods for preserving the ideal fluid balance in a variety of beverages.

This book excels in meal planning, advising on how to balance meals for the best nutrition, and provides helpful snacking suggestions specific to ileostomy patients. Taking on obstacles head-on, the author provides advice on recognizing and treating food intolerances as well as useful replacements for foods that cause issues. Active lifestyle choices are promoted as essential elements of a comprehensive strategy for ileostomy diets, including the inclusion of exercise for general well-being and stress management.

This book also addresses the pragmatic aspects of everyday living by providing information on simple-to-digest cooking techniques and a selection of meals designed with ileostomy dieters in mind. Strategic guidance on how to communicate dietary demands effectively is addressed when navigating social situations, especially eating out. The significance of routine health examinations is emphasized, along with advice on modifying the diet as appropriate.

This book "Proactive Approaches on Ileostomy Dieting" ends with an outlook on long-term success, inspiring readers to mark significant junctures along the way and strive toward creating a long-lasting, healthful lifestyle. In addition to providing readers with important information, this book's upbeat and engaging tone empowers them and points them in the direction of a proactive, happy life after ileostomy.

CHAPTER ONE

OVERVIEW OF ILEOSTOMY
Knowing About Ileostomy Surgery

An artificial incision called a stoma is made in the abdominal wall during ileostomy surgery, a medical technique that brings a section of the small intestine to the skin's surface. When there are problems with the lower portion of the digestive system, such as inflammatory bowel disease, colorectal cancer, or other disorders that affect the colon, this operation is frequently required. The ileostomy's function is to divert waste and stool from the rectum and colon and send them straight to the stoma.

Ileostomy surgery patients may feel a variety of feelings, such as anxiety and concern about how the procedure may affect their day-to-day lives. People must have a thorough awareness of the surgical procedure, possible side effects, and any necessary post-operative modifications. An expert surgeon skillfully diverts the small intestine during ileostomy surgery, creating a stoma that needs to be cared for carefully to avoid problems and infections.

Getting used to new routines and practices is part of adjusting to life with an ileostomy. Patients need to be taught how to change the ostomy pouch, take care of their stoma, and deal with any problems that may arise, like skin irritation. Navigating the physical and emotional elements of living with an ileostomy requires support from medical professionals, ostomy nurses, and support groups.

Diet is Important for Ileostomy Recovery

A patient's recovery and continued care after an ileostomy depends greatly on their diet. Following ileostomy surgery, the digestive system experiences major changes, so people need to be careful about what they eat to aid in recovery and avoid complications. The adjustment of the diet to account for the changed digestive process is one of the main factors. An ileostomy bypasses the colon, which means that the body has less time to absorb nutrients and water. For this reason, hydration and nutrient intake are essential for a full recovery.

Following surgery, patients are usually recommended to begin with a low-fiber diet and progressively introduce different foods to determine their tolerance levels. By taking a step-by-step approach, people can discover items that might irritate or cause blockages, which makes it possible for them to develop a diet plan that works for them. Hydration is crucial because people need to drink more liquids to stay well hydrated due to increased fluid loss via the stoma.

Patients with ileostomies must ensure that their intake of vital nutrients, including vitamins and minerals, is balanced. A well-rounded diet is ensured by including a range of foods, such as fruits, vegetables, and lean proteins. People may need to exercise caution while consuming high-fiber foods, though, as this may result in increased stool production. It's also critical to keep an eye out for symptoms of dehydration, electrolyte imbalances, and any side effects from particular foods.

In summary, having a thorough grasp of ileostomy surgery and the role nutrition plays in the healing process enables people to take charge of their health. Patients can improve their general well-being and look forward to a full life after ileostomy surgery by managing the physical and mental adaptations that come with the procedure and by taking a conscious approach to diet.

CHAPTER TWO

FUNDAMENTALS OF NUTRITION AND DIGESTION
An Overview Of The Digestive System

The body uses the digestive system, a sophisticated network of organs and functions, to process food and absorb nutrients for energy. It's important to know the fundamentals of digestion, particularly for those who have had an ileostomy, a surgical surgery that creates a stoma by redirecting the small intestine through an incision in the abdominal wall. To maintain optimal nutrition and health, people must modify their food habits due to this alteration in the digestive anatomy.

When food is eaten and combined with saliva that contains enzymes that begin breaking down carbs, digestion starts in the mouth. After passing down the esophagus and into the stomach, where the gastric fluids further break down proteins, the partially digested food exits the stomach. The semi-liquid mixture leaves the stomach and goes into the small intestine, which is where most of the absorption of nutrients takes place. The bulk intestine absorbs the remaining undigested material and forms feces as a result of the absorption of water and electrolytes.

When someone has an ileostomy, their normal digestive route is changed. A large amount of nutrients that are normally absorbed by the small intestine are instead sent toward the abdominal wall through the stoma. This alteration affects how some nutrients are absorbed, requiring dietary changes to ensure enough intake of nutrients.

Needs for Nutrition After an Ileostomy:

Individuals who have had ileostomy surgery experience particular difficulties in satisfying their nutritional demands. Changes in the small intestine affect the absorption of water, electrolytes, and some vitamins and minerals. This is a critical area for nutrition absorption. To maintain optimum health and well-being, an active approach to ileostomy dieting is therefore necessary.

The risk of dehydration after ileostomy is one of the main issues. Fluid loss through the stoma increases when the small intestine is diverted because less water is absorbed. People must stay properly hydrated by drinking enough fluids throughout the day. Color and frequency of urination might be helpful indicators of one's degree of hydration.

Moreover, the way essential nutrients like vitamin B12, iron, and electrolytes are absorbed may be impacted by the changed structure of the digestive system. Nutritional therapy following ileostomy care must include regular blood level monitoring and supplementation if needed. Meeting dietary needs can also be facilitated by including foods high in essential nutrients, such as leafy greens, lean meats, and fortified cereals.

The health of the digestive system also depends on dietary fiber, however, ileostomy patients must use caution when consuming large amounts of it. Insoluble fibers have the potential to enhance stoma output, even if soluble fibers are usually well tolerated. Maintaining gut health and managing potential problems can be accomplished by selecting easily digested, low-residue foods and balancing fiber consumption.

To sum up, a proactive strategy for ileostomy eating includes addressing particular dietary demands and gaining a thorough understanding of the modified digestive system. People with ileostomies can improve their general health and nutritional status by making dietary adjustments to maintain hydration, account for alterations in nutrient absorption, and regulate fiber intake.

CHAPTER THREE

LAYING A STRONG FOUNDATION: NECESSARY NUTRIENTS
Fats, Carbohydrates, and Proteins:

The three main macronutrients that are necessary for an ileostomy patient's general health and well-being are proteins, carbs, and fats. These nutrients are essential for the body's energy production, tissue repair, and metabolic processes. Comprehending the importance of consuming these macronutrients in a balanced manner is essential for ileostomy patients to prevent nutritional deficits and promote optimal health.

For ileostomy patients in particular, proteins are crucial because they promote tissue regeneration and repair, preserve muscular mass, and aid in the healing process. A well-rounded diet can benefit from the inclusion of high-quality protein sources such as lean meats, poultry, fish, eggs, and plant-based proteins like lentils and tofu. However, people who have an ileostomy should be aware of their tolerance levels because some foods high in protein can cause digestive problems.

As the main source of energy, carbohydrates supply the fuel required for daily tasks. Patients with ileostomies should concentrate on eating complex carbs, which include whole grains, fruits, and vegetables, to guarantee a steady release of energy and avoid abrupt changes in blood sugar levels. Since certain forms of carbs may be more quickly absorbed than others, it is important to balance your intake of carbohydrates to prevent potential problems like diarrhea.

For ileostomy patients, including healthy fats in the diet is equally important. Fats are involved in the synthesis of hormones, the absorption of nutrients, and general cell function. Choosing unsaturated fat sources, such as olive oil, avocados, nuts, and seeds, can support heart health and offer a concentrated energy source. It's important to keep an eye on fat intake because too much of it might cause loose stools and other digestive problems for those who have an ileostomy.

In conclusion, ileostomy patients must maintain a balanced diet that contains the right amounts of lipids, proteins, and carbs. Customizing dietary intake to meet tolerances and preferences guarantees that these macronutrients will have a good impact on both ileostomy maintenance and general health.

Minerals and Vitamins for Patients with Ileostomies:

Minerals and vitamins are essential for maintaining an ileostomy patient's health and energy. These patients must concentrate on a nutrient-rich diet to prevent deficits and enhance general well-being because of the altered intestinal landscape. The secret to creating a proactive dietary management strategy for ileostomy patients is to comprehend the particular vitamins and minerals that are essential.

Because they are fat-soluble, vitamins A, D, E, and K must be adequately absorbed from the diet. The modified digestive process of an ileostomy may make it difficult for an individual to absorb these vitamins.

It becomes crucial to include foods high in these vitamins, such as fatty fish, eggs, leafy greens, and dairy products that have been fortified. Deficits must be avoided by regular monitoring and, if required, supplementation under the supervision of medical professionals.

Water-soluble vitamins are essential for energy metabolism, neuronal function, and the production of red blood cells. These include the B-complex vitamins (B1, B2, B3, B6, B12, folate, and pantothenic acid).

Ileostomy patients should prioritize sources such as whole grains, lean meats, nuts, seeds, and fortified cereals to provide an adequate intake of these essential nutrients.

For ileostomy patients, minerals like calcium, magnesium, potassium, and salt must be carefully considered while making dietary choices. Making thoughtful food choices is crucial since malabsorption problems can affect the balance of minerals in the body.

Lean meats, leafy greens, nuts, seeds, dairy products, and fortified plant milk can all help to keep mineral levels at their ideal levels.

Ileostomy patients must collaborate extensively with medical specialists to evaluate and track their specific dietary requirements. Frequent blood work and consultations can help pinpoint particular deficiencies and direct the right supplementation or dietary changes.

By eating a range of nutrient-dense meals on a proactive basis, people with ileostomies can preserve good health and lower their risk of nutritional imbalances.

CHAPTER FOUR

ADAPTING YOUR DIET TO YOUR REQUIREMENTS
Tailoring Meal Plans for Patients with Ileostomies:

People who have ileostomies encounter particular difficulties that call for a customized approach to meal planning. A thorough awareness of the digestive modifications brought on by an ileostomy is necessary to modify one's diet to meet the unique requirements resulting from this surgical surgery.

Patients undergoing ileostomy have either all or part of their colon removed, rerouting the small intestine to a hole in the abdominal wall. To guarantee proper nutrition absorption, minimize dehydration, and manage any problems, a planned dietary approach is necessary due to this modification in the digestive tract.

Focusing on easily digestible foods is essential when creating customized diet regimens for ileostomy patients. The colon is essential for absorbing water and electrolytes, therefore maintaining fluid balance must be carefully managed in its absence. The danger of electrolyte imbalances and dehydration can be reduced by including foods that are easy on the digestive tract, such as well-cooked vegetables, lean meats, and easily digested grains. Moreover, distributing meals throughout the day in smaller servings can facilitate nutrition absorption effectively and avoid overloading the digestive tract.

Another important component of a customized diet for ileostomy patients is balancing their consumption of fiber. A certain amount of fiber is necessary for healthy digestion, but too much fiber can cause blockages in the small intestine's constricted area. As a result, people who have an ileostomy might benefit from starting with a low-fiber diet and introducing fiber-rich foods gradually to determine their tolerance levels. Patients can determine what kinds and quantities of fiber their digestive systems can tolerate without experiencing discomfort or problems by following this methodical technique.

Apart from managing the intake of fiber, it is imperative to keep an eye on specific compounds. For instance, some ileostomy patients may find it harder to handle foods that are spicy or heavy in fat. Including easily digested fats in the diet and steering clear of overly spicy foods might help promote general digestive comfort. Additionally, maintaining a food journal can be an invaluable resource for pinpointing particular triggers or intolerances, allowing people to customize their diets according to their reactions to various foods.

It takes continuing cooperation with medical professionals to create individualized food programs for ileostomy patients that can adjust to changing health conditions. Dietary recommendations can be adjusted based on a patient's changing needs with the guidance of a dietitian or other healthcare expert, ensuring that the diet continues to promote general health and well-being.

Foods to Love and Stay Away From:

After having an ileostomy, navigating the culinary landscape requires making deliberate decisions regarding the things one consumes regularly. For those who have an ileostomy, accepting some foods and shunning others becomes essential to preserving digestive health, averting problems, and guaranteeing general well-being.

Simple-to-digest and high in nutrients are the foods to include in an ileostomy-friendly diet. Fish, poultry, and tofu are examples of lean proteins that supply vital amino acids without overtaxing the digestive system. veggies that have been cooked, particularly those that have been well-cooked and peeled, provide vitamins and minerals without the difficulties that come with raw or fibrous veggies. In a similar vein, consuming quickly broken-down grains like refined pasta and white rice can give you energy without aggravating your digestive system.

On the other hand, it's important to steer clear of some meals to keep ileostomy patients comfortable and free from difficulties. Whole grains, nuts, seeds, and some raw vegetables are examples of high-fiber foods that can be difficult for the digestive system to process, which might result in obstructions in the small intestine's constriction. Foods that cause gas and carbonated drinks can cause bloating and discomfort, so it's best to avoid them altogether.

Furthermore, it might be advantageous for those who have an ileostomy to consume fewer hot and high-fat foods. These foods may be more difficult to digest and irritate the digestive tract, which could lead to discomfort or exacerbate pre-existing digestive problems. Preservatives and additives in processed foods should also be handled carefully because certain people may be allergic to them.

A diet that is ileostomy-friendly emphasizes the importance of hydration, and people are urged to stay well-hydrated all day. Dehydration can be avoided by drinking enough water, especially since the digestive system's ability to absorb water is diminished without the colon. To maintain general digestive health, it's crucial to make sensible beverage choices, such as drinking water, herbal teas, and other non-carbonated, non-caffeinated drinks.

In summary, careful consideration of dietary choices can greatly improve the quality of life for those who have an ileostomy. People can customize their diets to fit their specific demands and advance general well-being by embracing meals that are high in nutrients and easily digested while avoiding those that could cause digestive system problems. For those who have an ileostomy, continuous support is ensured via proactive diet modifications based on individual reactions and routine consultation with medical personnel.

CHAPTER FIVE

HYDRATION TECHNIQUES
The Significance of Hydration for Ileostomies

For those who have had an ileostomy—a surgical incision in the belly used to redirect the small intestine—hydration is essential to their health. Maintaining general health and avoiding potential ileostomy-related issues requires an understanding of the significance of hydration in this situation.

People who have had ileostomy surgery notice changes in their digestive systems, which causes more fluid to leak through the stoma. If this increased fluid flow is not properly managed, dehydration may ensue. Significant hazards associated with dehydration include electrolyte imbalances, renal impairment, and poor healing. Therefore, to avoid these issues and support the body's regular physiological processes, it is imperative to maintain adequate levels of hydration.

Furthermore, maintaining enough fluids is crucial for the digestive system's optimal operation and the avoidance of conditions like constipation. People who have an ileostomy must watch their fluid intake since they may be more vulnerable to dehydration as a result of increased fluid loss. Keeping an eye on the color and frequency of urine as well as responding to the body's thirst cues are essential components of ileostomy patients' hydration management.

People who have an ileostomy should take a proactive hydration strategy, taking into account variables including weather, level of physical activity, and general health. Creating a customized hydration regimen in conjunction with medical specialists guarantees that patients may satisfy their unique fluid requirements and preserve their best possible health following ileostomy surgery.

Drinking Different Beverages to Stay Hydrated:

After ileostomy surgery, it takes more than just water to stay well hydrated; a careful and varied approach to fluid intake is needed. Water is an essential part of any hydration plan, but adding other drinks can improve the whole experience and help people with ileostomies achieve better health results.

The possibility of electrolyte imbalances brought on by increased fluid production is one of the difficulties experienced by people who have an ileostomy. Sports drinks can be helpful in this situation since they replenish electrolytes lost via the stoma in addition to providing water. To prevent potential problems like diarrhea or excessive calorie intake, it's imperative to select low-sugar or sugar-free solutions.

Herbal teas and diluted fruit juices can be useful additions to the hydration arsenal, in addition to water and sports beverages. Natural sugars and extra nutrients can be obtained from diluted fruit juices, while herbal teas are a tasty and calorie-free substitute for regular water. Juices low in fiber should be carefully selected to reduce the possibility of digestive system obstructions.

Moreover, adding transparent soups and broths to the diet might help increase vitamin and hydration intake. These fluids can be especially helpful when there is considerable fluid loss or when recuperating from surgery because they are quickly absorbed by the body. But people should be careful not to overindulge in highly salted broths because too much sodium might cause dehydration.

In summary, the key to meeting the specific needs of people with ileostomies is to vary the sources of hydration for them. Through the integration of diverse beverage options and customization to individual dietary needs and preferences, patients can optimize their overall hydration regimen and foster improved outcomes for their health following ileostomy surgery.

CHAPTER SIX

ORGANIZING YOUR MEALS FOR ILEOSTOMY SUCCESS
Meal Timing to Get the Best Nutrition

For those with an ileostomy, achieving appropriate nutrition is a crucial component of meal planning. An ileostomy's effects on the digestive system might affect how well nutrients are absorbed, therefore maintaining a well-balanced diet is crucial. Including a range of dietary groups is essential to giving the body the nutrients it needs for general health and well-being.

Making sure you're getting enough protein is one of the main things to think about. For those with an ileostomy, protein is essential for both maintaining muscle mass and repairing damaged tissue. To satisfy protein requirements, incorporate lean meats, poultry, fish, eggs, dairy products, and plant-based protein sources like tofu and lentils. Consuming a variety of carbs, such as those found in fruits, vegetables, and whole grains, also contributes to digestive health by providing necessary dietary fiber and energy.

Keeping an eye on fat consumption is another essential component of meal planning for ileostomy success. Although good fats are necessary for the absorption of nutrients, too much fat can cause digestive problems. Choosing foods high in avocados, nuts, seeds, and olive oil—sources of good fats—can support a balanced diet without placing an excessive amount of strain on the digestive tract.

Furthermore, maintaining gut health is greatly aided by enough water, particularly for those who have an ileostomy. Due to the increased fluid loss through the stoma, dehydration is a significant problem that can be avoided by maintaining adequate hydration.

Maintaining fluid balance involves eating meals high in hydration, such as fruits and vegetables, and drinking lots of water throughout the day.

In conclusion, combining a range of nutrient-dense foods, monitoring healthy fat consumption, paying attention to protein intake, and making sure you're getting enough water are all important parts of meal balancing for optimal nutrition. It is crucial to tailor the diet to each patient's tastes and tolerances to proactively manage the nutritional demands of ileostomy patients.

Snacking Guide for Patients with Ileostomies

When eaten mindfully and about the health of your digestive system, snacks may be a useful and enjoyable part of an ileostomy diet. Making sensible snack selections can assist people with ileostomies sustain their energy levels, avoiding nutritional shortages, and promoting their general well-being.

For ileostomy patients, selecting easily digestible snacks is essential. Refined grains, well-cooked veggies, peeled and prepared fruits, and low-residue foods can all help reduce the likelihood of upset stomachs. Adding readily digested protein sources, like cheese, nut butter, or yogurt, can further enhance the nutritional value and satisfaction of a snack.

When it comes to snacking, portion control is another crucial factor for ileostomy patients. Smaller, more frequent snacks throughout the day can aid in better nutrient absorption and digestion load management in place of larger meals. Yogurt cups, chopped fruits, and almonds are a few examples of pre-portioned snacks that might be handy for controlling portion amounts.

Additionally, snacking should be a chance to mix up the diet and include a variety of nutrients. A well-rounded nutritional profile can be achieved by including a variety of food groups, such as fruits, vegetables, lean meats, and healthy fats. Snacking can be made more pleasurable and fulfilling by experimenting with different flavor combinations and textures.

For ileostomy patients, time is just as important as food selection when it comes to snacking successfully. Snacking in between meals, as opposed to either before or right after, helps the digestive system break down food more quickly. Establishing a nutritious snacking practice can be facilitated by paying attention to the body's signals and eating when hungry.

In conclusion, careful meal selection, portion management, diversity, and timing are key components of successful ileostomy snacking. People who have an ileostomy can have a nutritious, well-balanced diet that meets their specific digestive requirements by including these snacking suggestions into their overall meal plan.

CHAPTER SEVEN

NAVIGATING CHALLENGES: DEALING WITH FOOD INTOLERANCES
Identifying and Managing Food Intolerances:

Managing the difficulties brought on by food intolerances is essential to continuing an active ileostomy diet. For people who have an ileostomy, it is critical to recognize and understand particular food intolerances because they have a direct impact on their digestive system and general health.

Keeping a thorough food journal, recording not only what is eaten but also how the body reacts, is an essential part of this process. Identifying patterns of bloating, irregular bowel movements, or pain can shed light on possible dietary intolerances. Accurately identifying particular intolerances and interpreting these trends requires speaking with a certified dietician or healthcare practitioner.

Diets based on elimination are frequently used to identify problematic items. Through a methodical elimination and eventual reintroduction of specific food groups, people can monitor their bodies' responses and pinpoint triggers. diets known to create gas, raw vegetables, and high-fiber diets are common offenders for ileostomy patients. Although it can take some time, the elimination process is essential to developing a customized and successful diet plan.

Medical tests can also yield useful information. Examples of these procedures include breath tests for carbohydrate malabsorption and allergy testing. These tests provide a complete picture of a person's unique food intolerances when paired with the data from the food diary and elimination diet. Designing a diet that guarantees the best possible nutrient absorption without jeopardizing intestinal health requires an understanding of this.

In conclusion, treating food intolerances in ileostomy patients necessitates a multifaceted strategy that includes medical tests, expert advice, and sometimes even personal observations. For those who have an ileostomy, a customized meal plan can greatly improve overall quality of life by fostering comfort in the digestive system and general health.

Changing Out Troublesome Foods:

A crucial tactic in the proactive treatment of ileostomy dieting is the substitution of troublesome foods, which enables people to stick to a nutritious and balanced diet while avoiding triggers that could aggravate their condition or create digestive problems. Because of the nature of an ileostomy, some foods may be restricted, therefore it's critical to identify suitable substitutes to ensure a balanced and fulfilling diet.

Ileostomy patients frequently struggle with the restriction of high-fiber diets. Although fiber is important for digestive health in general, it might cause blockages or excessive output in people who have an ileostomy. People can address this by using low-residue alternatives in place of conventional high-fiber sources. Selecting well-cooked and peeled fruits and vegetables or going for white rice instead of brown rice, for instance, might help lower the fiber content while retaining vital nutrients.

When lactose intolerance is detected, it's important to identify dairy products that work well as alternatives. Thankfully, there are several lactose-free substitutes out there, such as soy milk, almond milk, and lactose-free yogurt. These substitutes not only offer the essential nutrients present in dairy products but also shield the digestive tract from the discomfort caused by lactose intolerance.

Furthermore, since some protein sources might be difficult to digest, ileostomy patients may need to modify their protein intake. Selecting protein sources that are lean and easily absorbed, such as fish, chicken, and eggs, can assist satisfy dietary requirements without overtaxing the digestive system.

To sum up, switching out troublesome meals is a proactive and flexible way to manage ileostomy dieting. A gratifying and nutritionally balanced diet that promotes general health and well-being can be made by individuals by finding appropriate options and making educated decisions.

CHAPTER EIGHT

ACTIVE LIFESTYLE SELECTIONS
Including Exercise in Ileostomy Diets for General Well-Being:

One of the most important aspects of proactive approaches to ileostomy dieting is maintaining an active lifestyle. Although it makes sense that people who have an ileostomy might be wary of exercising, physical activity is essential for maintaining general health. Frequent exercise has positive effects on mental and emotional well-being in addition to physical health.

Developing a customized fitness regimen can improve energy levels, improve cardiovascular health, and aid with weight control—all critical components of successfully managing an ileostomy. Walking, swimming, and cycling are examples of moderate aerobic exercises that can be especially helpful without putting too much strain on the stomach region. Exercises that strengthen the muscles in the core can also help support the abdominal wall and lower the risk of problems.

Exercise also improves mental health by lowering stress and worry that are frequently brought on by life alterations, like having an ileostomy. Exercise releases endorphins, which are the body's natural mood enhancers and promote optimism. Additionally, it offers a chance for social engagement, which fosters a sense of support and community.

It is advised that people who have an ileostomy speak with medical experts or certified trainers to create individualized training regimens that take into account their particular requirements and restrictions. Individuals who have an ileostomy can actively improve their general health and lead active, satisfying lives by making exercise a regular part of their daily regimen.

Managing Stress During an Ileostomy Diet:

Recognizing the complex relationship between the mind and body, proactive methods for ileostomy dieting are based on effective stress management. People who have an ileostomy frequently deal with certain difficulties that can raise their stress levels. These difficulties include worries about their nutrition, how they look, and possible lifestyle changes. Putting stress management techniques into practice is crucial for advancing mental and physical well-being.

The development of mindfulness techniques is a crucial component of stress management. Being mindful entails accepting ideas and feelings without passing judgment on them and being in the present. By encouraging calmness and mental clarity, methods like yoga, meditation, and deep breathing techniques can assist people with ileostomies manage stress.

These activities improve general mental health in addition to lowering stress.

Creating a strong support network is another essential part of stress management. Making connections with people who have gone through comparable struggles, participating in support groups, or enlisting the help of loved ones can offer consolation and insightful information.

Positive emotional environments are influenced by relationships that are strengthened and understanding that is fostered via open communication about feelings and concerns.

Participating in enjoyable and soothing hobbies can also help lower stress levels. In addition to providing a welcome diversion, hobbies, pastimes, and artistic endeavors support a more contented and balanced way of life. Individuals who have an ileostomy can enhance their overall well-being by adopting a proactive and comprehensive approach to stress management.

This will enable them to face the difficulties associated with nutrition and lifestyle modifications with courage and optimism.

CHAPTRE NINE

RECIPES FOR PATIENTS WITH ILEOSTOMIES
Simple Cooking Techniques:

When it comes to ileostomy diets, proactive approaches take great care to prepare meals that are both mild on the digestive tract and easily absorbed. It's critical to give priority to cooking methods for ileostomy patients that reduce irritation or discomfort. Steaming is a great option since it makes food simpler to digest while preserving its inherent flavors and nutrients. With vegetables, this technique is especially helpful since it guarantees their tenderness and ease of digestion.

Poaching is another suggested cooking method, particularly for meats like fish or fowl. Food is poached by slowly cooking it in liquid to keep it wet and from drying out or becoming too rough.

This technique improves the dish's palatability while also being soft on the stomach. Pasta and grains can also be prepared successfully by simmering and boiling. These methods make it possible to cook food thoroughly without using a lot of fat or oil, which helps people with ileostomies digest food more easily.

Cooking techniques like roasting and grilling can be used sparingly, paying attention to the doneness level. Although these techniques can improve food flavors, they may need to be used sparingly to prevent extremely harsh textures that could be difficult for the digestive system to process. Meats can be made more palatable for ileostomy patients by marinating them before cooking.

Another proactive measure is to include fermented foods in the diet. Certain food ingredients are broken down by fermentation, which facilitates better digestion. Fermented foods like sauerkraut, kefir, and yogurt can help create a diet that is both nourishing to the digestive system and well-balanced. All things considered, selecting cooking techniques that are simple to digest is critical to maintaining the health of ileostomy patients since it guarantees that they get the nutrients they need without unduly taxing their digestive systems.

Recipes Designed with Ileostomy Dieters in Mind:

Nutrient density and careful ingredient selection are key when developing recipes for ileostomy dieters. Lean meats, poultry, and fish are examples of easily digestible proteins that should be included. Essential amino acids are supplied by these proteins without taxing the digestive system excessively. Herbs and spices can be used to enhance the flavor of baked fish or grilled poultry without introducing too much fat or irritants.

A well-balanced diet for ileostomates must include a range of vegetables in recipes. Choosing vegetables that are easily digested and well-cooked, such as spinach, zucchini, and carrots, guarantees a good dose of vitamins and minerals without causing problems for your digestive system. A side dish of mashed potatoes with a small quantity of butter or olive oil can be a satisfying and simple meal.

While whole grains are a good source of fiber and energy, people with ileostomies might benefit more from refined grains. Refined flour products such as white rice, pasta, and bread can be added to recipes to offer carbohydrates without raising the risk of constipation. It's critical to keep an eye on each person's tolerances and modify the fiber intake accordingly.

It's important to choose desserts that are readily digestible and minimal in fat. Desserts made with fruit, such as poached pears or baked apples, can sate a sweet taste without going overboard. Desserts with yogurt or gelatin can also be included to offer variation and ease of digestion.

In conclusion, foods designed with ileostomy dieters in mind should emphasize refined grains, low-fat sweets, well-cooked veggies, and readily digestible proteins. These dishes are meant to be tasty and nutritious, taking into account the special requirements of people who have ileostomies.

CHAPTER TEN

DINING OUT AND SOCIAL OCCURRENCES
Techniques for Eating Out While Having an Ileostomy

Eating out might be difficult at first for people who have an ileostomy, but with proactive measures, people can still enjoy social events without sacrificing their comfort or health. Developing a strategic attitude is essential when perusing restaurant menus. A good strategy is to do your homework ahead of time and find eateries that offer a wide variety of menu items and can accommodate particular dietary requirements. Many contemporary restaurants offer online menus, which let patrons carefully review ingredient lists and select meals that are in line with their post-ileostomy diet.

Also, it's crucial to communicate with the restaurant staff. It's best to subtly let servers know that you have an ileostomy and assist them in understanding the necessary dietary adjustments and limits. Proactively discussing the components used in each dish with the chef can guarantee better knowledge and allow for customized alterations. It is powerful to adopt an assertive ordering style, and restaurants frequently value customers who are unambiguous in communicating their wants.

Making choices that are simple to understand is another crucial tactic. Choosing foods that are soft, cooked through, and free of fibrous materials will facilitate digestion and reduce the possibility of problems. Safe options include cooked veggies, grilled or steamed proteins, and easily digested grains. Portion control can also be helpful because it helps lessen the stress on the digestive system and prevent overeating.

For individuals with ileostomies, meal timing is very important. Arranging dinner dates when people are more energetic can improve the whole experience. Proactive scheduling can lead to enhanced comfort, better digestion, and a greater capacity to enjoy the meal.

Proactive eating tactics essentially consist of careful preparation, clear communication, and thoughtful meal selection. People who have an ileostomy can participate in social events with confidence and without sacrificing their nutritional needs if they follow these procedures.

Effectively Communicating Dietary Needs

A key component of effectively managing an ileostomy in social settings is communicating dietary demands. Encouraging and understanding interactions with friends, family, and hosts require open and honest communication. Cooperation and empathy are enhanced when you inform people close to you about the intricacies of your post-ileostomy diet, such as food limitations or the requirement for frequent, smaller meals.

It's critical to discreetly and confidently disclose dietary requirements at social events. One way to foster understanding is to gently explain dietary constraints and show gratitude for the hospitality you have received. It can also make things easier for the person with an ileostomy and their hosts if you offer to help with meal preparation or bring a dish that complies with your dietary needs.

Effective communication between wait staff and chefs is critical in restaurants. It's critical to communicate the significance of avoiding particular products or cooking techniques clearly and succinctly. It can also help to avoid needless agony or humiliation to quietly provide information regarding the ileostomy.

A medical alert card or bracelet can also be a preventative precaution, giving vital details regarding the ileostomy and dietary requirements in an emergency. This tool can be especially helpful in medical emergencies where timely and accurate information is critical or in situations where verbal communication may be difficult.

People with ileostomies can comfortably handle social settings by prioritizing good communication, which in turn fosters understanding and support from others in their immediate vicinity. People can enjoy social contact without jeopardizing their health in a more inclusive and accommodating atmosphere created by open communication and preemptive efforts.

CHAPTER ELEVEN

OBSERVING AND MODIFYING: FREQUENT CHECK-INS
The Value of Continual Health Evaluations

For those who have an ileostomy, routine health exams are essential since they are critical to preserving general health. These evaluations offer insightful information about the person's health and enable prompt identification of any possible problems or consequences. Consistent health check-ins allow patients and healthcare providers to keep an eye on important health indicators like overall digestive health, hydration status, and nutritional levels in the context of proactive approaches to ileostomy management.

Early detection of dietary deficiencies is one of the main advantages of routine health examinations. Patients with ileostomies may be more susceptible to specific dietary deficits because of altered digestion and absorption processes. Healthcare professionals may closely monitor the body's levels of vital vitamins and minerals through routine examinations, which enables prompt dietary modifications or supplementation.

In addition, health evaluations give patients and medical professionals a forum for candid conversation. People can talk about any difficulties or worries they have with their ileostomy diet in this continuing conversation and get tailored advice. Better long-term outcomes are promoted by encouraging a proactive approach to healthcare, where possible problems can be addressed before they worsen.

Regular health evaluations play a crucial role in assessing the state of hydration in addition to nutritional considerations. For those who have an ileostomy, staying properly hydrated is essential because increased fluid loss might happen through the stoma. Healthcare professionals can evaluate hydration levels and offer suggestions to enhance fluid consumption through routine check-ins, guaranteeing adequate hydration and averting issues linked to dehydration.

In general, it is impossible to overestimate the significance of routine health examinations in the context of proactive strategies for ileostomy nutrition. These evaluations function as a preventative measure to preserve good health, identify possible problems early, and promote a cooperative and encouraging connection between medical staff and patients.

Making Dietary Changes as Necessary:

A key component of proactive ileostomy diet strategies is diet adaptation and modification. People who have an ileostomy frequently deal with particular difficulties with stoma maintenance, nutrition absorption, and digestion.

To meet the body's changing needs and advance general well-being, a dynamic and adaptable approach to food choices is necessary.

An important factor to take into account while modifying a diet is a person's reaction to particular meals. People who have an ileostomy may react differently to some foods, which could cause discomfort, alter the consistency of their stools, or even cause blockages. People who regularly self-monitor and are aware of these reactions are better able to recognize trigger foods and make judgments about whether to limit or avoid eating them.

Furthermore, diet modifications are essential for controlling the stoma's output consistency. To control the consistency of their stools and reduce the possibility of issues like blockages or discomfort around the stoma site, people may need to adjust the amount of fiber they consume in their diet.

Individuals and medical experts must work together to customize dietary suggestions to each person's unique needs and tolerances.

Sometimes medical conditions, surgeries, or drug changes can necessitate dietary changes. For instance, some drugs may affect how well nutrients are absorbed, requiring dietary changes to guarantee sufficient consumption. Healthcare providers can help people make these changes by providing knowledge about dietary needs and the ideal ratio of macro and micronutrients.

Making dietary changes also requires keeping up with the latest findings, medical developments, and recommended procedures for ileostomy care. People who get this continuous education are better equipped to make educated food decisions and stay up to date on the most recent advancements in stoma care and nutrition.

To sum up, dietary modifications constitute a dynamic and unique part of proactive ileostomy treatment.

It entails an ongoing process of self-monitoring, working together with medical professionals, and keeping up with the most recent developments in stoma care and nutrition. By guaranteeing that people can modify their diets to suit their evolving demands, this strategy promotes optimum health and a high standard of living.

CHAPITRE TWELVE

DEVELOPING A SUCCESSFUL LONG TERM
Honoring Significant Achievers in Ileostomy Diet

Being an ileostomy patient means that dieting must be proactive, and long-term success depends on marking progress along the route. The process of adjusting to an ileostomy includes learning about one's body, adjusting one's food, and striking a balance that supports one's mental and physical health.

The ability to identify trigger foods is a crucial step in the ileostomy diet. Maintaining a thorough food journal is crucial for monitoring the impact of various foods on the digestive tract. When people who have an ileostomy experiment with different foods, they can rejoice when they figure out which ones cause pain or digestive problems.

With this knowledge, people can make more educated decisions that improve their quality of life and general health.

Maintaining appropriate hydration is another accomplishment to be proud of. People who have ileostomies may be more susceptible to dehydration because of increased fluid loss through the stoma. A significant accomplishment is forming routines that guarantee a sufficient intake of fluids, such as eating foods high in water and drinking water mindfully. Marking this achievement not only shows appreciation for the work required to maintain hydration but also emphasizes the benefits to general health and wellbeing.

In managing ileostomy care, achieving nutritionally adequate and well-balanced food is a major accomplishment. This entails supplying the body with a range of nutrient-dense foods to guarantee it gets the vitamins and minerals it needs. Honoring the capacity to design a diet that promotes maximum health cultivates a favorable rapport with food and reaffirms the notion that maintaining an ileostomy does not entail sacrificing nutritional value.

It's vital to celebrate not just the food gains but also the emotional fortitude gained along the way. Living with an ileostomy can have a significant psychological impact, and recognizing the strength one gains from overcoming obstacles is essential to long-term success. Marking achievements in ileostomy dieting goes beyond material gains; it also acknowledges the holistic approach required for a happy and meaningful life.

Constructing a Healthful and Sustainable Lifestyle

It takes more than just diet to create a sustainable and healthy lifestyle for those with ileostomies. It covers a wide range of strategies, such as social interactions, mental health, and physical exercise. Creating such a lifestyle improves the quality of life overall and makes a substantial contribution to long-term success.

Including regular physical activity is a crucial component of a sustainable lifestyle. Exercise improves general well-being, helps people maintain a healthy weight, and reduces stress in addition to its physical health benefits. People who have ileostomies should investigate activities that suit their tastes and talents, adapting as necessary. Celebrating accomplishments in physical activity, such as hitting a fitness target or maintaining a regular exercise schedule, serves to emphasize the value of continued physical activity for long-term health.

Stressing mental health is just another essential element of a healthy way of living. It can be difficult to deal with the emotional issues of having an ileostomy, therefore long-term success depends on making mental health a priority. A resilient mindset is influenced by activities like mindfulness, meditation, and getting help from mental health specialists. Honoring mental health achievements, such as conquering emotional obstacles or implementing healthy coping strategies, highlights the significance of a comprehensive approach to health.

Having social ties is essential to creating a sustainable and healthful lifestyle. A strong support network is established through participating in support groups, making connections with people who have gone through similar things, and cultivating friendships and familial ties. Celebrating social interaction milestones—like making deep relationships or engaging in engaging activities—highlights the value of a strong support system in assisting individuals in overcoming the obstacles associated with living with an ileostomy.

Furthermore, creating a sustainable lifestyle requires taking a proactive stance on self-care. This entails going to the doctor regularly, keeping up with new advancements in ileostomy care, and speaking out for oneself. The significance of being proactive in preserving optimal health is reinforced when self-care accomplishments are celebrated, such as regularly following a medical regimen or proactively addressing possible problems.

In conclusion, creating a sustainable and healthful lifestyle for those who have an ileostomy requires a multifaceted strategy that takes into account their social, emotional, and physical health. In addition to honoring accomplishments, marking life's major events serves to reaffirm the tenacity and resolve required for long-term success with ileostomy care.

www.ingramcontent.com/pod-product-compliance
Lightning Source LLC
Chambersburg PA
CBHW070803290526
45795CB00002B/611